YOUR KNOWLEDGE HAS VALUE

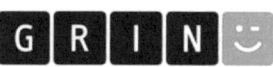

Bibliographic information published by the German National Library:

The German National Library lists this publication in the National Bibliography; detailed bibliographic data are available on the Internet at http://dnb.dnb.de .

Imprint:

Copyright © 2016 GRIN Verlag, Open Publishing GmbH
Print and binding: Books on Demand GmbH, Norderstedt Germany
ISBN: 978-3-668-17521-1

This book at GRIN:

http://www.grin.com/en/e-book/317184/the-theory-of-health-as-expanding-human-consciousness-margaret-newman-s

Fain Ayiera

The Theory of Health as Expanding Human Consciousness. Margaret Newman's Contribution to Nursing Theory and Practice

GRIN Publishing

GRIN - Your knowledge has value

Since its foundation in 1998, GRIN has specialized in publishing academic texts by students, college teachers and other academics as e-book and printed book. The website www.grin.com is an ideal platform for presenting term papers, final papers, scientific essays, dissertations and specialist books.

Content

Abstract

A nursing theory is a name that refers to a body of knowledge that is utilized in supporting nursing. It is also a framework for knowledge that is organized and it describes various nursing phenomena at a specific and concrete level. It consists of sets of concepts, relationships, definitions, prepositions, and definitions that are borrowed from models of nursing. In this assignment, we are going focus on the theory of Margaret Newman, its impacts and influence in the current field of nursing and its applications in the various clinical setting. We will check the background of the nurse theorist and her contribution to the nursing field.

Introduction

Margaret Newman is a nursing theorist who is recognized for the Theory of Health Expanding Human Consciousness. She was born in the year 1933 in Memphis Tennessee. She was raised in a Christian family because she was brought up in Baptist church where her mother was working as a secretary. Being brought in a Christian setting environment, it motivated her to join the missionary service later in her life. While in the mission, she realized that she was in no position to help people spiritually without taking care of them physically. She remembered that she had a nursing student roommate in her college, and she thought of taking that path for herself so that she could go back and help the people physical needs. She returned home after receiving news that her mother was ill. Her mother was suffering from chronic irreversible health condition which was amyotrophic lateral sclerosis. She decided to take care of her mother and become her primary care giver (Newman, 1990). It's during that time that she realized that being diagnosed with a chronic disease does not make one unhealthy. She was so much convinced that her mother could still experience healthiness despite being diagnosed with the disease. She was able to formulate the condition of her mother as being confined rather than being defined by it.

She also discovered that during the entire hardship process of the disease of nursing her mother, she also started experiencing the same symptoms and alterations in movement, time, consciousness and space (Fawcett et al., 2012). She developed great connectedness towards her mother, and they knew each other a deeper and a better way than the earlier times. This is the experience that motivated her to go back to school and study nursing to help others like her mother. Expanding consciousness theory was introduced as a nursing theory in the late 1970s.

This theory was developed through the study of its application cancer and cardiac disease between 1986 and 1997(Newman, 1990). The theory has evolved in the year 2010 to include the health of all people regardless of whether they have a disease or not (Newman, 1990; Fawcett., 2012).

Theory of Health as Expanding Consciousness

The theory of health expanding consciousness came from Rogers' theory of unitary human beings. The assumption of Rogers regarding the interaction of individuals with their environment is used as a basis of consciousness being a manifestation of patterns evolving from the environment-person relationship. Margaret defines consciousness as an informational capacity of the system (human being) that is, the system ability to interact with the surrounding (Fawcett et al., 2012). Consciousness includes both the cognitive and the effective awareness that is usually related to consciousness and the interconnectedness of the whole living system. The information pattern which is the consciousness system is the larger part that is not a divided pattern of an expanding world.

She claims that each individual in every situation, regardless of how hopeless or disordered it may seem, takes part in the process of expanding the consciousness universally which is a process of one becoming oneself and discovering greater life meanings, and reaching new dimensions of connectedness with other individuals and the universe.

Contributions of Newman to the field of nursing

She was a trained nurse who assisted patients to recover and maintain their health. She was a lecturer in Minnesota University, and she taught nursing students from diverse backgrounds, and since she is role models, many nursing students have borrowed from her. She was the first to come up with the theory of health as expanding consciousness which was officially introduced as a nursing theory in the 1970s (Alligood, 2013). Her theory is of great use in the modern nursing profession because nurses and patients are using it today. She applied her nursing theory to help give better care to her patients (Butts et al., 2013).

Assumptions

Health encompasses conditions such as diseases or pathology in medical terms. Another assumption is that the conditions of pathology can be considered as a sign of the patient's total pattern. The third assumption is that each individual patient pattern that in time expresses itself as pathology is primary and it exists before functional or structural changes (Alligood, 2013; Butts et al., 2013).

Pathology removal will not change the individual pattern of the patient. If the only way for an individual pattern of the patient to express itself is through getting sick, then that is considered as the health of that particular individual patient. The final assumption is that an expansion of consciousness is, therefore, health (Stout et al., 2012).

According to this theory, health does not mean the absence of a disease or a process of becoming healthy after being sick. Nurses usually interact with such people: individuals facing debilitation, uncertainty about life, loss and eventual death related to chronic diseases. The theory has progressed, and it now considers the health of people regardless whether they have an illness or not. The theory emphasizes that every individual in each situation no matter how hopeless or disordered it may seem is part and parcel of the process of universal (Edgar et al., 2012).

The patients are constantly interacting with the universe and its energy because they are open in the universe energy system. The individual process pattern evolves each time because of the pattern of interaction. Nurses should be able to understand their patient's pattern because it is important (Noam et al., 2013). When we recognize the pattern, it means we are expanding consciousness. For a disease to be able to express itself, it depends on the individual pattern. Therefore, before the symptoms of illness appear, the pathology of the disease must exist first. Because of this, when the symptoms of an illness of an individual are removed, it does not change the structure of an individual structure (Stout et al., 2012).

Newman's redefines the process of nursing as using her nursing process of recognizing an individual in relation to their environment, and it involves understanding consciousness. A nurse can use power to create a higher level of consciousness when he/she understands his/her patients. Therefore, it assists nurses to know the process of the disease, its recovery as well as the ways for prevention. She tries to show the relationships between time, space and movement. The temporal patterns of the patient are the time and space, and these two are complementary to each other. A unique pattern of reality is shown through space and time because individuals keep on changing through the two (Fawcett et al., 2012).

This theory argues that disease and health are synthesized as health. That is joining the state of one being an, in this case, a disease with its opposite which is, the absence of a disease to give health. She considers human in her model as unitary. That means that human beings cannot be divided into parts and that they are inseparable from the larger field of unitary. Human beings are identified by their consciousness patterns (Alligood, 2013; Butts et al., 2013). That an individual does not possess consciousness but rather they are consciousness (Edgar et al., 2012). Individuals are centers for consciousness with a general pattern of consciousness expansion. She defines environment as a universe made up of open systems.

The wholeness of the person is identified by the use of pattern and it changes with time and becomes difficult to predict. The human environmental process is identified by pattern, and it is distinguished by meaning which is synonymous with pattern. Pattern change constantly with time and it is comprised of; - movement- space-time, rhythmic- basic movement and diversity-seen part. Movement: This can be either movement of matter, reception, self-awareness, a means of communicating and reality. Time can be subjective or objective. Space can either be the personal space or inner space.

Meaningful events and individual are discussed due to pattern recognition as they lived experiences are uncovered. Opportunities for new choices of life might turn up during the disorganization periods. A person can discover new opportunities for direction and action during the caring process. When good choices are made, increased connectedness, freedom, and relationship opportunities are made possible through human awareness and potential (Alligood, 2013).

From her model caring is the human health experience is nursing. She views it as a partnership between the patient and the nurse, with the involved parties glowing in the sense of higher consciousness levels.

Applications of the Theory to Nursing

This theory applies to modern nursing because of its emphasis on continuous care outside the clinical settings. The activities that support and improve the health of an individual can still be carried outside the health care centers. Therefore, there is need for empowerment and social support. Home based care assist to reduce the work load of the healthcare providers and lessens the economic burden of health care centers especially in the third world countries (Hek et al., 2013)

Some concepts in the theory are intrinsic factors in the nursing intervention for example time and movement. Motion range, ambulation, breathing, and coughing are parameters that are employed by nurses in practice. This theory can well be applied in patients who are diagnosed with disease such as cancer, HIV/AIDS among others. It can be devastating to individual when they are diagnosed with either of the named diseases. This can affect the family and the patients as well as they face emotional, spiritual and social stresses that affect the treatment response, lifestyle changes, home and work role disruption and stigma. These people face challenges by changes in their own mortality, self-image, sexuality and even the reproductive capacity. Nurses should assist the patients who are diagnosed either HIV positive or with cancer to know that each day of a person is precious and the life of a person is contained in that present moment (Stout et al., 2012). They should fight stigma and apply Newman's theory that being sick does not make one unhealthy.

One can be healthy and whole even after being diagnosed with a disease or with no disease (Alligood, 2013; Butts et al., 2013). Health is not the opposite of sickness but rather both are manifestation of the two. Initially, people used to hide an illness after being diagnosed HIV positive because of fear but nurses have proved to be of so much help by assisting these patients to expand consciousness around their illness. Therefore, nurses assist their patients in pattern recognition to make them understand new possibilities for action and that there is room for health in illness. The obligation of a nurse is to help their patients to realize that they have power within them that can help raise their level of consciousness (Edgar et al., 2012). Individuals today can accept their health status and thanks to Newman's theory. Elderly people in the nursing homes may experience diminished human connection but nurses working in the nursing homes use the Newman's theory to make their clients feel more connected. Therefore it is becoming easier to administer drugs and create a good nursing care plan. Expanding consciousness concepts assist nurses to care for their patients holistically (Alligood, 2013)

Influence of Margaret on My Personal / Professional Life

Studying Newman's background one realizes that she had passion for nursing and helping others. Spirituality and caring are complementary to improve health of an individual. When she joined missionary that physical care was also important and she joined school to study nursing so as to attend to her people well. With hard work and determination we can achieve our dreams. She is more than a nurse to me because she contributed globally to make nursing profession what it is today.

Conclusion

Newman's theory is considered as a grand nursing theory whereby she states that those individuals are indivisible. Heath is the core of this theory and it the process of creating awareness with the environment and one self. The work of the nurse to help their patient realize the power contained in them that can help them recover their health.

Reference

Newman, M. A. (1990). Newman's theory of health as praxis. *Nursing Science Quarterly, 3*(1), 37-41.

Fawcett, J., & Desanto-Madeya, S. (2012). *Contemporary nursing knowledge: Analysis and evaluation of nursing models and theories*. FA Davis.

Edgar, C., McRorie, M., & Sneddon, I. (2012). Emotional intelligence, personality and the decoding of non-verbal expressions of emotion.*Personality and Individual Differences, 52*(3), 295-300.

Alligood, M. R. (2013). *Nursing theorists and their work*. Elsevier Health Sciences.

Butts, J. B., Bandhauer, D., & Rich, K. L. (2013). *Philosophies and theories for advanced nursing practice*. Jones & Bartlett Publishers.

Noam, G. G., & Fischer, K. W. (2013). *Development and vulnerability in close relationships*. Psychology Press.

Stout, N. L., Binkley, J. M., Schmitz, K. H., Andrews, K., Hayes, S. C., Campbell, K. L., ... & Fabian, C. (2012). A prospective surveillance model for rehabilitation for women with breast cancer. *Cancer, 118*(S8), 2191-2200.

Hek, K., Demirkan, A., Lahti, J., Terracciano, A., Teumer, A., Cornelis, M. C., ... & Liu, Y. (2013). A genome-wide association study of depressive symptoms. *Biological psychiatry, 73*(7), 667-678.

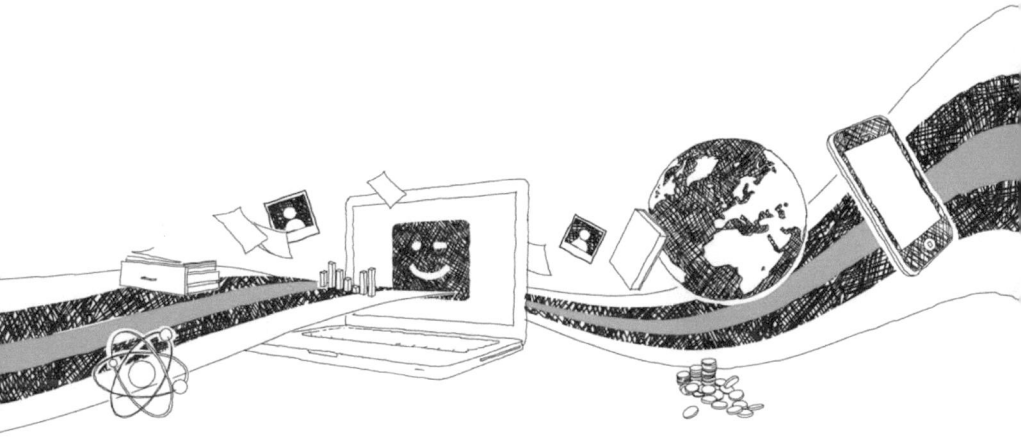
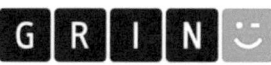